YOUR KNOWLEDGE HAS VALUE

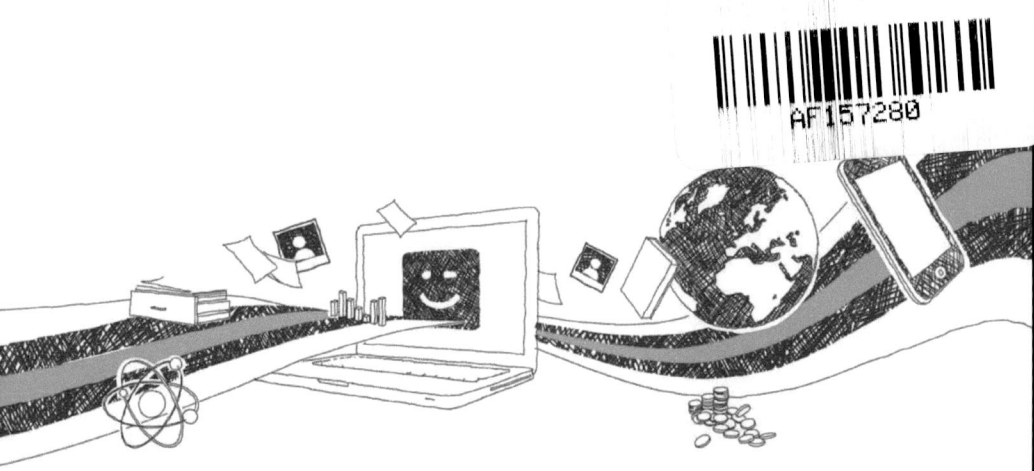

AF157280

- We will publish your bachelor's and master's thesis, essays and papers

- Your own eBook and book - sold worldwide in all relevant shops

- Earn money with each sale

Upload your text at www.GRIN.com
and publish for free

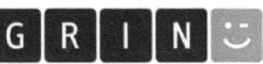

Bibliographic information published by the German National Library:

The German National Library lists this publication in the National Bibliography; detailed bibliographic data are available on the Internet at http://dnb.dnb.de .

Imprint:

Copyright © 2010 GRIN Verlag, Open Publishing GmbH
Print and binding: Books on Demand GmbH, Norderstedt Germany
ISBN: 9783640638932

This book at GRIN:

http://www.grin.com/en/e-book/152002/ontologies-and-electronic-health-record-related-standards

Stefan Schroeder

Ontologies and Electronic Health Record related Standards

GRIN Publishing

GRIN - Your knowledge has value

Since its foundation in 1998, GRIN has specialized in publishing academic texts by students, college teachers and other academics as e-book and printed book. The website www.grin.com is an ideal platform for presenting term papers, final papers, scientific essays, dissertations and specialist books.

Visit us on the internet:

http://www.grin.com/

http://www.facebook.com/grincom

http://www.twitter.com/grin_com

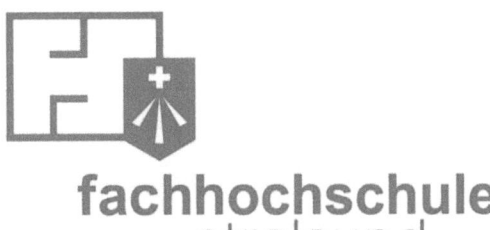

fachhochschule stralsund

university of applied sciences

fachbereich school of
elektrotechnik electrical engineering +
+ informatik computer science

Scientific research for the seminar
Electronic Health Record
At the master degree course Medical Informatics

Topic
Ontologies and EHR related standards

Vorgelegt am 11. Januar 2010 von
Stefan Schroeder

1. Introduction

1.1. Philosophical

"What is existence?" A question easy to ask, but hard to answer. Concerning these and other philosophical questions, Ontology is a matter of the theoretical philosophy. It tries to categorize and classify a given reality, in order to create a shareable schema of it. Contrariwise, this "reality" could be any kind of world or closed theme, for example a specific domain (cars, diseases) or a concept of use (language, network).

Philosophers tried to describe and analyze our known world. Their ambition was to find a way, to create relations between different aspects of reality and afterwards, to pull the revealed associations together. This offers a view onto reality, which contains the knowledge on the one hand, but also on the other hand, the comprehension of the knowledge. The target was to discuss the basic organization of entities and relations, which aims at the philosophers wanted ability, to have a complete and qualified view onto a domain (like reality, the largest domain of all).

The idea which started the invention and processing of ontology in the past was the willing of human to understand their position within their environment. *What is a thing? What is an attribute? What is existence* – and furthermore, *what things are said to be existing?* Still today, the answers to this questions are hard to find and strongly depending on the individuals' disposition.

1.2. Informational

In an informational way, ontology tries to category different information systems and put them into classification. Usually, information systems are inhomogeneous and cannot operate together (Figure 1). And as they share no common ontology, it is impossible to trade data between them.

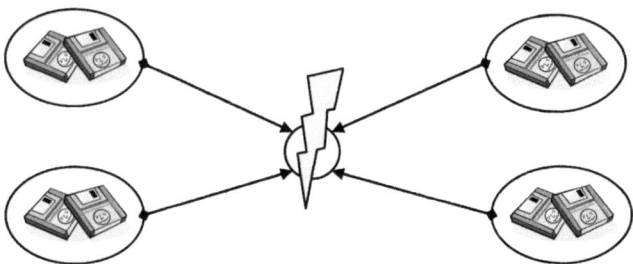

Figure 1: Impossible communication between different information systems [own work]

At this point, new technologies and conceptions are needed, because the communication of information systems is essential in modern IT solutions. Two problems need to be solved: at first, all involved parties have to use the same syntax, so that they are able to receive communicated data correctly. The next step is the correct interpretation of the shared information – does the information at the sender and at the receiver does have exactly the same meaning? This problem educed two possible solutions:

1. Build a translation from one system to another (Figure 2)

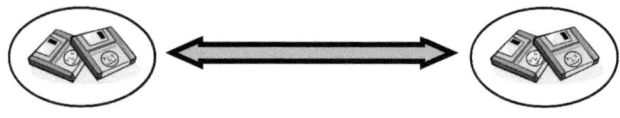

tion [own work]

This is a very easy-to-use technology, as there is only a need for one translation when connecting two different information systems. But as more information systems are getting part of the communication model, the number of translations growth by $\frac{n(n-1)}{2}$ (Figure 3).

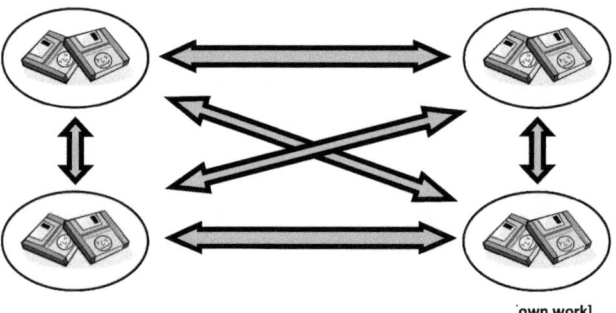

[own work]

That means every single party of the network needs a single connection to each other party. This network topology is called "fully connected" or "peer-to-peer".

2. In contrast, the second solution uses one central common used translation protocol – called conceptualization (Figure 4). This conceptualization could be an ontology, which holds all needed information about the involved communication system in order to enable transfer of information through it. Keep in mind, that not the technical/informational process is the problem, but the correct interpretation of the information.

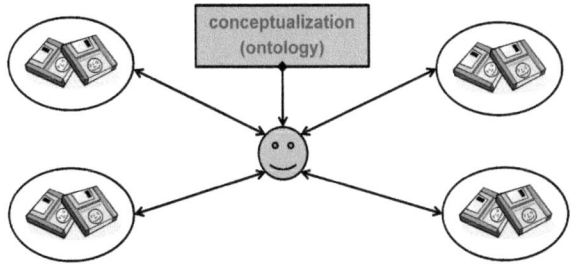

Figure 4: four connections and a common conzeptualization [own work]

This network topology could be compared to a „star" or „client-server-model".

These two solutions provide different advantages and disadvantages. At one hand, a client-server-model lowers the costs for installing the communication network, as there are much less connection needed than in peer-to-peer network (Chart 1).

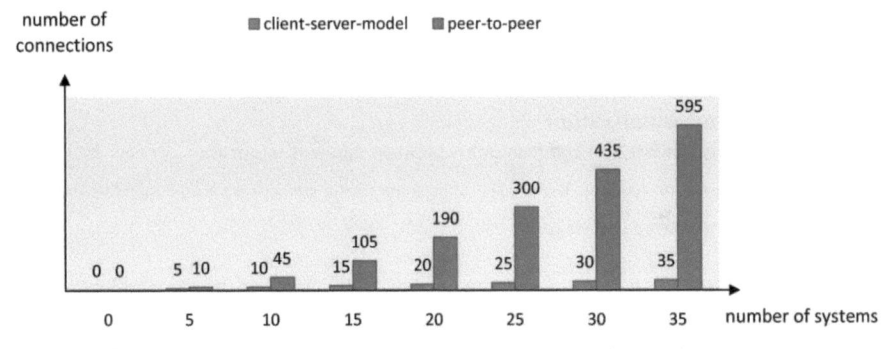

Chart 1: number of connections in relation to number of involved systems [own work]

Furthermore, adding new parties to the network is more efficient and easy as per each new client, just one new connection is needed (connection to the conceptualization). In a peer-to-peer network, one new client needs to be connected to every existing client and vice versa. Scaling a client-server network is also easier and cheaper than a peer-to-peer based one.

On the other hand, using a central communication solution provides some disadvantages. At first, the malfunction of a common used concept would have an impact on all parties and inhibit any kind of data transfer. At second, the dependency on a common used translation script could restrict or lower the informational capability of single party members. That means that clients with more modern or extensive communication protocols then the central communication concept are not able to utilize them – as they depend on the conceptual regulations of the central communication concept.

1.3. Biomedical

In healthcare related software, ontology enable communication between different parties that are involved in healthcare business, such as hospitals or health insurance companies (Figure 5).

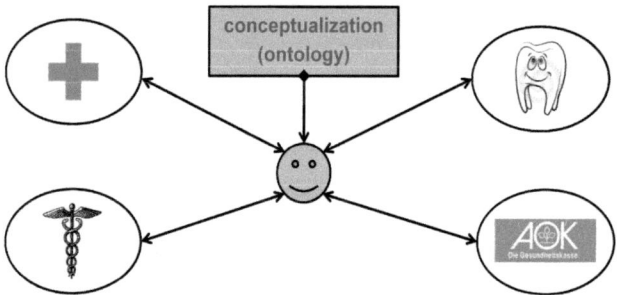

Figure 5: communication in health care related infrastructure [own work]

1.4. Conceptualization

As mentioned before, the communication between different information systems does require a specific translation concept. The process of creating such a concept is called conceptualization and a possible outcome is an ontology.

In other words, this outcome is an abstract and reduced view of your world, including all its objects and their relations to each other. Figure 6 shows a world, which consists of one table and five blocks. The objects that are part of the world are described in a set D:

$$D = \{a, b, c, d, e, table\}$$

The relations between these objects are described in a set R, containing the relations "on" (pair of bricks that stay on one another), "ontable" (bricks that are directly on the table) and "top" (bricks that are on top).

$$W = \begin{cases} on\ (a,b)(b,c)(d,e) \\ ontable\ (c,e) \\ top\ (a,d) \end{cases}$$

The concept of the world shown in Figure 6 is a tuple K.

$$K = (D, W)$$

As this is a quiet easy process, the problem of creating a concept occurs when the world changes (Figure 7).

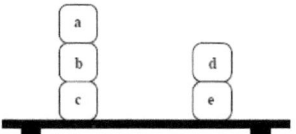

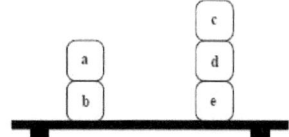

Figure 6: a world containing of a table and some blocks   **Figure 7: the same world with changed relations**

The concept K is not correct anymore and insufficient to describe the world in Figure 7 exactly. There is a need for a third component – a set of all possible versions of the world, called R.

$$K = (D, W, R)$$

The set R completes the triple K, which is now an adequate and accurate ontology that describes the domain "block world".

2. Technology

The previous chapter should give you an overview about the topic ontologies. In course of that, it comprised the different kinds of definitions about ontologies and it was shown how ontologies represent knowledge. That is the basic for the following chapters of this report. Now it is time to focus that topic somewhat more exactly. This chapter contains the domains semantic interoperability and ontology languages. It represents an important part of this work, because it shows the importance and advantages of ontologies on the one hand, as well as the structure and the various possibilities of implementation on the other hand. In the first part it is shown how ontologies can facilitate semantic interoperability between different systems. Subsequently, the different ontology languages are presented.

2.1. Semantic interoperability

Nowadays the term "semantic interoperability" is often used in several areas of information and communication technology, because today a coherent and standardized communication between many different systems is desired and necessary, too. Therefore semantic interoperability exists, if various systems can interact and make effective use of the terms are used in the interaction. The use of ontology is a useful approach to solution to reach that goal. For a more detailed description of this context it is useful to explain an example. A common project regarding to the topics ontologies and semantic interoperability is called "Semantic Web". It is the development of a standardized language for the description and structuring of Internet resources. The Semantic Web based on ontologies whereby search agents can realize a more effective search. If you want to search the word SOAP, e.g., through the whole WWW with the purpose to find something about a network specification, you will get many results concerning daily soaps and cleaning products as well. Of course, you can try to search with the terms "SOAP + network", but it makes it not more effective. Maybe you will get a few results which conform to your perceptions, however it is from disadvantage that there will be at least as many unwanted results.

The major profit of the Semantic Web is the independent decision making of the system. It ensures that all results you will get are applicable. This is made possible because ontologies consists of different classes which have a taxonomic hierarchy. Thus relations and instances the search agent have the ability to except all unnecessary meanings of a term (e.g.; "SOAP") It starts at a top level ontology class and becomes more detailed step-by-step. (e.g., technologies -> communication -> network -> protocols -> SOAP).

So the main goal is to make information about electronic resources machine-readable by adding semantic markups. That brings an indescribable benefit, because machines can interpret the data independently. In this way it is possible for agents to draw conclusions and recognize relations between different data. Thus resources can be found more purposefully and context-referred. The most important techniques of the Semantic Web are RDF (Resource Description Framework) as a standard for Metadata and XML (Xtensible Markup Language) as a markup language for data exchange. These terms will be envisaged in the next part of this work.

2.2. Ontology Language

Now we know which advantages the use of ontologies offers, but it is always a concept. A machine-readable language is needed to create such an ontology. Ontology languages are languages that comply with this requirement and thus a fundamental part of the Semantic Web. XML can be used for standardized data presentation on the web, but it cannot use to describe the interpretation of a text on the web and XML cannot show ontology specific features like instances, relations between classes and so on.

Resource Description Framework

The Resource Description Framework (RDF) is a formal language to provide meta data in the WWW. The Resource Description Framework was published for the first time in 1998 as a recommendation of the World Wide Web Consortium (W3C), but it was taken back for processing and completed in 2004.

The forerunner of RDF was the Meta Content Framework (MCF), which was developed by 1997. To describe more complex relationships between resources the RDF was expanded through RDF Schema expanded. The RDF Schema defines the vocabulary for a particular application and is based on the Ontology-principle. The RDF Schema is similar to the DTD for XML documents and import sets the Syntax firm. The RDF Schema is based on a set-theoretic class model, which allows establish a formal semantic description of the used RDF elements. [6]

There are two ways to display the description of the meta data. A graphical model (Figure 8) and an XML based syntax (below Figure 8).

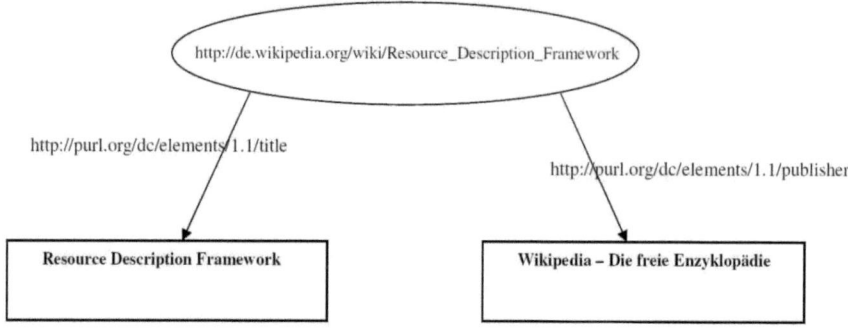

Figure 8: short example as a graphcial model [7]

same example in RDF Schema:

```
<?xml version="1.0" encoding="UTF-8" ?>
<rdf:RDF xmlns:rdf="http://www.w3.org/1999/02/22-rdf-syntax-ns#"
    xmlns:dc="http://purl.org/dc/elements/1.1/">
  <rdf:Description rdf:about="http://de.wikipedia.org/wiki/Resource_Description_Framework">
    <dc:title>Resource Description Framework</dc:title>
    <dc:publisher>Wikipedia – Die freie Enzyklopädie</dc:publisher>
  </rdf:Description>
</rdf:RDF>
```

In this case it is shown how to use RDF to depict the relation between an article, the title and the editor based on Dublin Core[1]. (= metadata-scheme to describe documents [8]).

The Resource Description Framework lacks important features such as cardinalities and transitive, inverse or symmetric properties. Furthermore, RDF admits inferences and conclusions only to a limited extend due to the lack of standard Semantic. Therefore, two successors have been developed for RDF: OIL which was developed by European researchers and DAML-ONT which has been developed in the USA. Later both projects joined into DAML + OIL and further developed through the Joint EU / US Committee on Agent Markup Languages. This gave DAML + OIL to the World Wide Web Consortium (W3C) as the basis for a standard. The W3C formed the Web Ontology (webont) Working Goup which developed the Web Ontology Language based on DAML + OIL.

Web Ontology Language (OWL)

The Web Ontology Language (OWL) is a recommendation of the W3C and supported so-called Description Logics. Description Logic is equivalent to a decidable subset of first-order logic. OWL allows ontologies to create the basis of a formal description, these messages are also machine read- and interpretable.

```
<owl:Ontology rdf:about=""/>
<owl:Class rdf:ID="Gender"/>
<owl:Class rdf:ID="Person"/>
<owl:Class rdf:ID="Woman">
 <rdfs:subClassOf rdf:resource="#Person"/>
 <owl:equivalentClass>
  <owl:Restriction>
   <owl:onProperty rdf:resource="#Gender"/>
   <owl:hasValue rdf:resource="#female" rdf:type="#Gender"/>
  </owl:Restriction>
 </owl:equivalentClass>
</owl:Class>
<owl:ObjectProperty rdf:ID="gender" rdf:type="..." >
...
</owl:ObjectProperty>
<owl:DatatypeProperty rdf:ID="name" rdf:type="...">
...
</owl:DatatypeProperty>
<owl:DatatypeProperty rdf:ID="firstname" rdf:type="...">
...
</owl:DatatypeProperty>
<Person rdf:ID="STilgner" firstname="Susanne" name"Tilgner">
<Gender rdf:resource="#female"/>
</Person>
```

This OWL example describes the concepts <Person>, <Gender> and <Woman>. A Woman is defined as a <Person> with the value <female> include in property <gender>. The property has to associate to the class <Gender>. For this reason the instance <STilgner> is described as <Person> a Woman, because the value is female [9].

There are three different types of OWL: OWL Lite is a easy to implement subset of OWL OWL DL is a combination of the Web Ontology Language and Description Logics (DL) with a few restrictions to ensure the presentability. OWL Full matches with OWL DL without the restrictions. However, this implies that the ontologies are not decidable. It is unlikely that any reasoning software will be able to support complete reasoning for OWL Full.

3. Ontology in EHR Standards

Before the report addresses ontology in EHR standard, the author wants to remind, that ontology always is a model of reality and contains all its objects and relations. In contrast, the EHR standards using models of information – called archetypes. These information models contain only knowledge that is important for the special medical actions. The main task is related to the question: what information should be captured? E.g. a blood pressure measurement consists of diastolic, systolic and pulse information. On the opposite, blood pressure ontology tries to answer the question, what exactly a blood pressure is – concerning anatomy, physics, units of measurement etc.

In humans' view of the world, a single piece of information is always a part of reality. As archetypes are models of information and ontology reflects a real world, archetypes are also a part of ontology. In regard to EHR software, this means that on the one side the software tries to collect information. On the other side, the EHR software access clinical archetypes that are based on ontology. In other words: archetypes could be referenced to ontology (Figure 9).

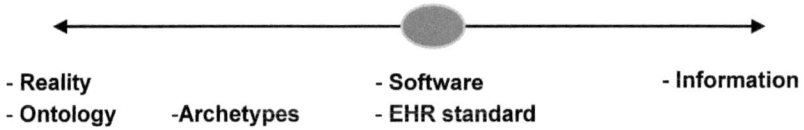

| - Reality | | - Software | - Information |
| - Ontology | -Archetypes | - EHR standard | |

Figure 9: relation between reality, software and information [own work]

Today, the standard EN13606 and the openEHR software use the archetype definition language (ADL), which includes an "ontology header". The ADL is known as a formal language to describe information models, which could be referenced within a patient record (for example, an archetype for blood pressure measurement). Finally, the ontology header holds data constraints and terminological bindings.

But the ontology header does not provide full semantic interoperability or semantic operations; it contains only definitions of terms and data. Furthermore, there is one ontology for one standard – nut no common used ontology (Figure 10).

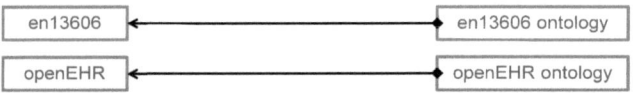

This paper demonstrates two solutions to solve this problem. At first, the use of an integrated ontology seems useful [4]. The two different ontologies are mapped to an integrated ontology that is used by both standards.

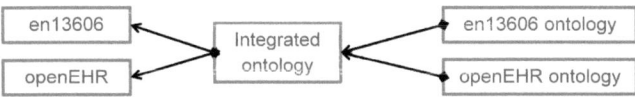

Even if there is still use of the archetype definition language, the information models are based on the same ontology and would share the same binding and constraints. Unfortunately, this does not support semantic operations anyway.

The second solution is called "ontology-based archetype transformation process" [5]. Based on a shared ontology, the EN13606 and openEHR archetypes are transformed from the ADL into the web ontology language (OWL). This new OWL archetypes are able to be processed by semantic operations like comparison or classification. Furthermore, this new archetypes would allow semantic interoperability between the openEHR and EN13606 systems.

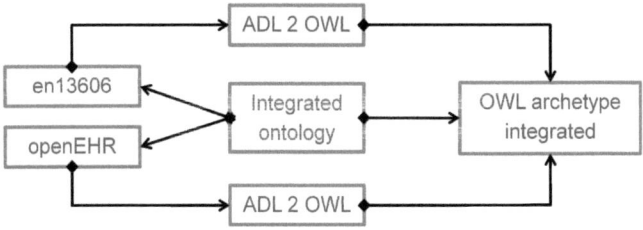

Figure 12: ontology-based archetype transformation process [own work]

4. Further Development

4.1. Mapping

As ontology is very often a concept for a specified domain, more than one ontology could exist for the domain. Ontology bases communication fail, when different ontologies are used within one communication network. To prevent problems or disadvantages caused by multiple concepts, the mapping became essential. An example was shown in *ontologies in EHR standards*, where the EN13606 and openEHR ontology are containing knowledge about the same domain (healthcare), but where not compatible in use.

During a "mapping process", two ontologies are merged together. Source ontology one (O_{S1}) and source ontology two (O_{S2}) result in the target ontology (O_T).

$$O_{S1} + O_{S2} = O_T$$

Logical, this mapping process contains of three steps:

1. analyze of both ontologies to get information about objects and relations
2. find identical objects and relations
3. create an output ontology, where identical relations & objects are melt together, and unequal ones are separated

Figure 13 and Figure 14 are showing two different ontologies ("Creature" and "Living Thing"), which contain a concept for the same domain (categorize an individual). But there slight differences between both ontologies, which causes a lack of interoperability if two information systems are based on these different concepts.

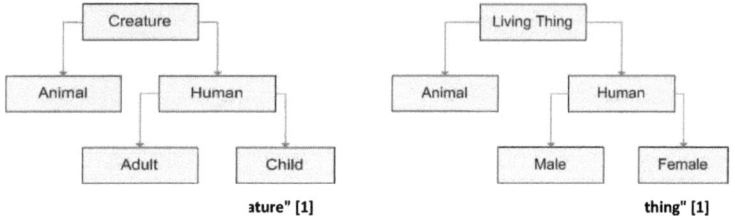

ature" [1]   thing" [1]

After the mapping process, the target ontology should contain the knowledge of both source ontologies - including all relations (Figure 15).

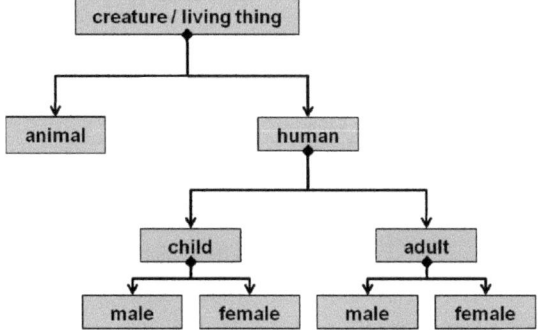

Figure 15 illustrates how the target ontology contains the two source concepts. The top level node, now combines the "creature" and "living thing" entity. Furthermore, the relation "child"/"adult" to "human" (Figure 16) and the relation "male"/"female" to "human" (Figure 17) are merged from two different two-level-models to one three-level-model.

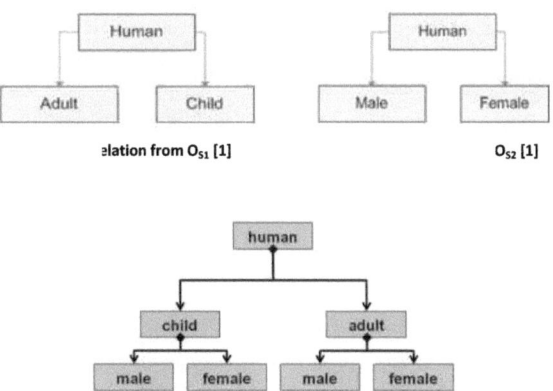

Figure 18: relation from O_T [own work]

The process of mapping two different ontologies is quiet complex and highly time-consuming. There are a few technologies to automate the mapping, like the language to specify mappings between ontologies from the university of insbruck [1] or the chimaera ontology environment from the Stanford University [2].

This report addresses another solution provided by the Stanford University, called PROMPT: Algorithm and Tool for Automated Ontology Merging and Alignment" [3]. It is a semi-automatic merge progress of two ontologies, which is based on their class names. PROMPT makes suggestion how to map the different classes, while the users input decide whether the suggestions were correct or wrong.

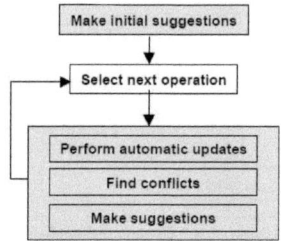

Figure 19: the flow of PROMPT algorithm [3]

Figure 19 shows the workflow. After PROMPT made an initial suggestion, the user needs to accept or reject the suggestion. Afterwards, PROMPT analyze the interactions in order to detect conflicts within the target ontology. If so, PROMPT again needs user interaction to solve the problem. If not, other suggestions are performed and the ontology mapping process continuous.

PROMPT was implemented as an extension to Protégé-2000, the latest in a series of knowledge-acquisition tools developed in the Stanford laboratories. Protégé-2000 uses direct-manipulation techniques for ontology editing and allows users to add new features by using plug-ins[3].

Human experts followed 90% of PROMPTs suggestions and 75% followed the "conflict-resolution strategies" [3]. Contra wise, the developers of PROMPT admitted that they chose relatively small and uncontroversial source ontologies. But in contrast to other merging tools (like Chimaera), PROMPT offers the user possibilities what to do if an error or conflict occurs (conflict-resolution strategies) [3].

4.2. eHealth application

For applications in Healthcare it may be a high benefit to use ontologies. A few years ago the SNOMED-CT was published which represent a big amount of information concerning terms in medicine. The development of OWL 1.1 eliminated one of the most significant barriers to use of OWL for SNOMED, since it permits the identification of tractable sublanguages capable of handling the size and complexity of SNOMED (Kent Spackman, 2007). The NHS in UK started a £6.2 billion "Connecting for Health" IT program. The key component is Care Records Service (CRS), which allows interactive patient record services accessible 24/7 access to patient information [10].

Local service providers store the detailed records and diverse applications support radiology, pharmacy, etc. The applications exchange messages containing semantically rich clinical information. The SNOMED-CT ontology provides common vocabulary for data. SNOMED-CT comprised about 1.000.000 terms associated with over 400.000 concepts, thus it is much larger than most available OWL ontologies [9]. The NHS version extended to 542.380 classes with 19.828 additional named classes and 148.821 class drug taxonomy (primitive hierarchy) [12].

Another project in France concerned with self-medication. Many people die due to wrong self-medication year after year. The system provides on-line advices. It will be made available to 20 million customers of French health insurance companies.

Patients have their own simple health care record (SEHR) and the diagnosis system considers symptom descriptions, SEHR, Q&A and self-medication KB. An OWL reasoner advice on treatment and check for contra-indications, adverse-drug-reaction, etc [13]. One possible decision could be that the patient do not take the drug x if he or she suffers from y. It could leads to the side-effect z. Figure 20 displays the whole approach of the self-medication application. The data is taken from various drug terminologies, e.g. European Pharmaceutical Market Research Association (EphMRA) or Anatomical Therapeutic Chemical (ATC).

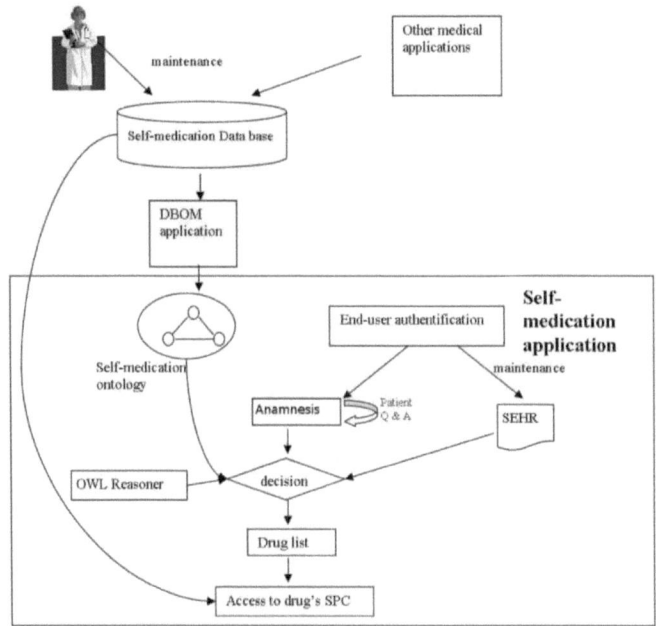

Figure 20: Self-medication application [13]

There are also interesting areas of application beyond the healthcare sector. The expert system POPS is used by NASA to find the experts and employees for certain subjects and tasks. A total of up to seven distributed databases, which contains the data about employee training, experiences, projects and much more, are scanned with POPS. From the existing database an RDF ontology was created, which serves as the basis for the application. To build up a connection to the experts it was implemented "Social Network" Visualization [13].

References

[1] A Language to Specify Mapping Between Ontologies (Franc¸ois Scharffe, Jos de Bruijn) from the Digital Enterprise Research Institute

[2] The Chimaera Ontology Environment (Deborah L. McGuinness, Richard Fikes, James Rice, Steven Wilder from the Stanford University, Stanford, CA

[3] PROMPT: Algorithm and Tool for Automated Ontology Merging and Alignment (Natalya Fridman Noy and Mark A. Musen) from the Stanford University, Stanford, CA

[4] Towards ISO 13606 and openEHR Archetype-Based Semantic Interoperability (Catalina Martínez-Costa, Marcos Menárguez-Tortosa, J. T. Fernández-Breis) from the Universidad de Murcia, CP 30100, Murcia

[5] Ontology-based Archetype Interoperability and Management (Catalina Martínez-Costa, Marcos Menárguez-Tortosa, J. T. Fernández-Breis) from the Universidad de Murcia, CP 30100, Murcia

[6] World Wide Web Consortium: Resource Description Language (http://www.w3.org/RDF)

[7] Wikipedia – Die freie Enzyklopädie: Resource Description Framework, (http://de.wikipedia.org/wiki/Resource_Description_Framework)

[8] Wikipedia – Die freie Enzyklopädie: Dublin Core, (http://en.wikipedia.org/wiki/Dublin_core)

[9] Wikipedia – Die freue Enzyklopädie: OWL, (http://de.wikipedia.org/wiki/Web_Ontology_Language)

[10] NHS Care Records Service, (http://www.nhscarerecords.nhs.uk/)

[11] "Is Semantic Web technology ready for Healthcare?" (http://ftp1.de.freebsd.org/Publications/CEUR-WS/Vol-194/paper2.pdf)

[12] "Semantic Web Landscape 2009", (http://www.slideshare.net/LeeFeigenbaum/semantic-web-landscape-2009)

[13] "Semantic Web Technologies in Practice", (http://clarkparsia.com/talks/semweb-tech-in-practice/)

List of figures

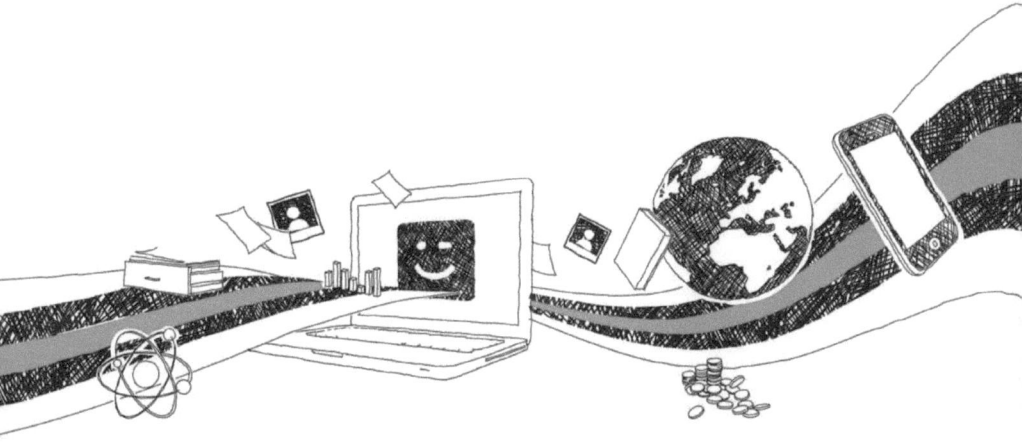
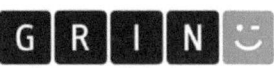

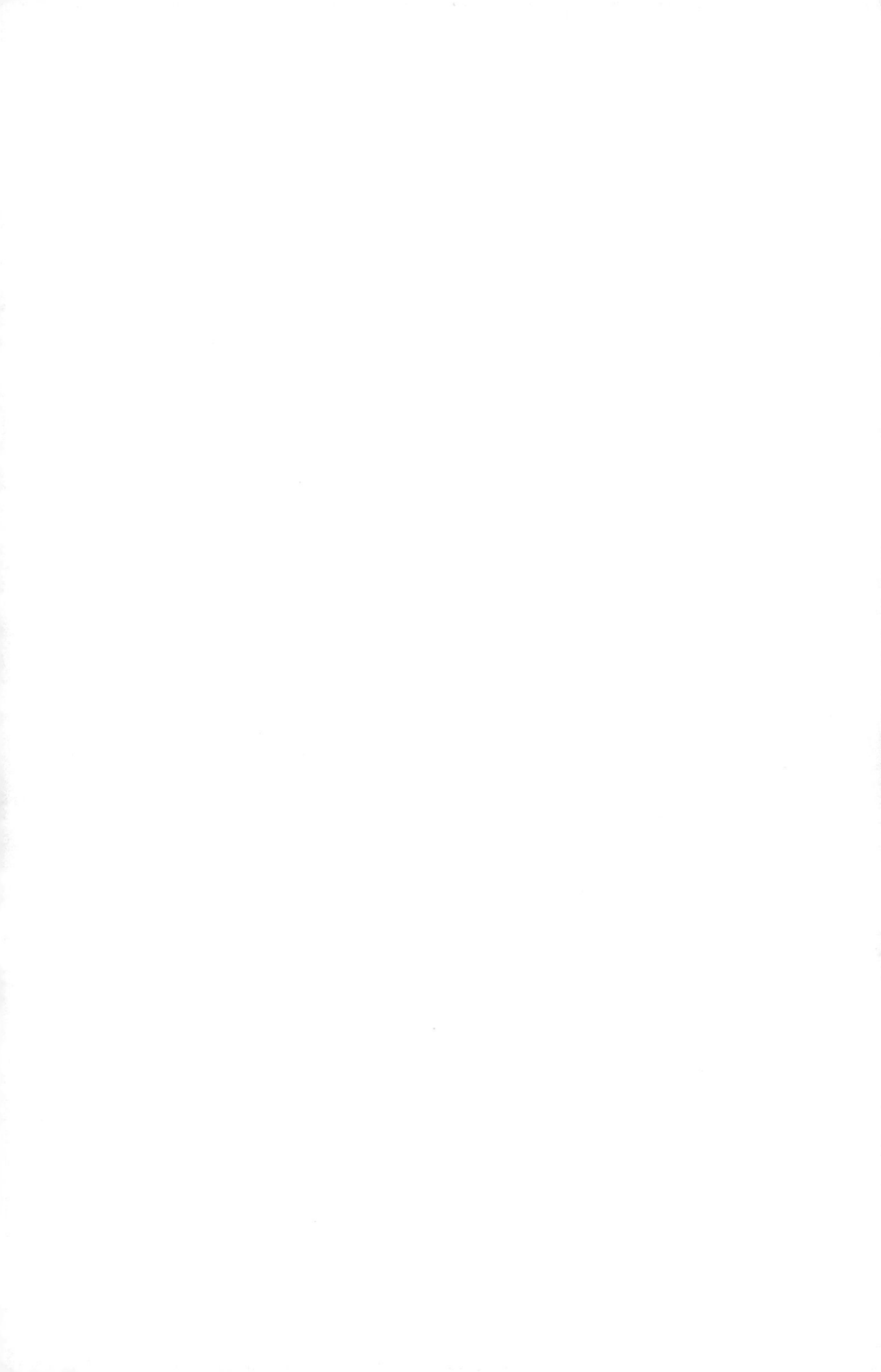